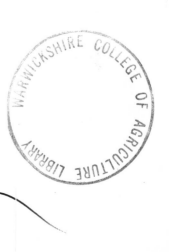

THE TREATMENT OF HORSES
BY ACUPUNCTURE

THE TREATMENT OF HORSES BY ACUPUNCTURE

By
DR. MED. VET. ERWIN WESTERMAYER

Translated by
DR. AC. D. LAWSON-WOOD, F.Br.Ac.A.,

&

J. LAWSON-WOOD, Ph.D.

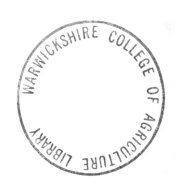

THE C.W. DANIEL COMPANY LTD
1, CHURCH PATH, SAFFRON WALDEN
ESSEX, ENGLAND

First published in Great Britain in 1979
by Health Science Press,
Bradford, Holsworthy, England

Reprinted 1985

Originally published in Germany
under the title *Atlas der Akupunktur
des Pferdes* in 1976 by
WBV Biologisch-Medizinische Verlagsgesellschaft mbH & Co., KG,
7060 Schorndorf, Ipfweg 5, Germany

ISBN 0 850 32161 1

Printed in Great Britain by Whitstable Litho, Whitstable, Kent.

Contents

6

Foreword

Nearly ten years ago, when I began to include acupuncture in my veterinary practice as a treatment method, there were but few publications available in German on veterinary acupuncture (JÖCHLE, LAMBARD, KOTHBAUER, GREIFF, etc.). In those days the only published works were on acupuncture applied to human beings, so I had to delve into these and try to translate human acupuncture-point positions into terms of animal anatomical structure, thus discovering the points for myself. Although this was very difficult, owing to the different anatomical structure of our domestic animals, I was able to locate a number of points for a useful range of symptoms. These first efforts were confined to a limited range of symptoms such as Lameness and Facilitation of Labour.

In recent years interest in acupuncture has grown in the western world. Attempts to establish this method in the service of veterinary medicine have found expression in publications on animal-acupuncture (KOTHBAUER/Austria, YOUNG/USA, OKADA-MEIYN, etc.).

My own experiences, intensive study of all publications available to me, and daily practical applications have convinced me that acupuncture can be used in veterinary medicine as an additional method having a vast therapeutic potential.

It was with considerable scepticism that I looked at the first translations from the Chinese (as an example of treatment obtainable—a picture of a horse's flanks overprinted with points together with a description of the position and of the symptoms applicable to each point.). It was true I knew that for centuries acupuncture had had its place in China's veterinary medicine, nevertheless the citing of indications such as tetanus for acupuncture treatment elicited in a western trained veterinary doctor only an uncomprehending shaking of the head. However, it was actually through these apparently non-sensical indications that I saw something happen which made me decide to go more deeply into acupuncture.

A few years ago I was confronted with a case of a horse in an advanced state of tetanus. It stood rigid, as good as no longer able to move itself at all, suffering from lock-jaw, etc., so that I wanted to put the animal down to save it from an agonizing end. However, at the request of the animal's owner, I made a further attempt at therapy with serum, antibiotics against secondary infection, remedies containing curare, and sedatives; but all was of no avail. Then I remembered that the Chinese give acupuncture points for tetanus. At the outset I must make it clear that I did not bring the suffering moribund patient through with acupuncture, but the needling which I did had a result that I would not have thought possible. Within a minute of needling six points on the head a muscle quivering took place throughout the whole of the horse's body, and the animal which before could not move laid its forequarters on the manger. It remained a whole day more able to move but not able to take in food.

In describing this I do not, of course, imply that I can confirm the correctness of the tetanus indication. Also, thanks to preventive inoculation, lock-jaw diseases seldom occur. But the fact that at such an advanced stage the musculature was activated through needle stimulation and the animal's pain relieved compels reflection.

In the course of years I have seen similar astonishing results with a whole lot of other symptoms. Nevertheless I have not considered veterinary acupuncture as a possible sole therapy, but I have always tried to incorporate it into our modern therapeutic armament as an auxiliary therapy. I am convinced that as an auxiliary therapy, acupuncture can offer valid additional help often achieving results not otherwise obtainable. It goes without saying, of course, that correctly applied it is a harmless technique.

In offering this work on acupuncture treatment of horses. I am only too aware that I can in no way put forward any claim whatsoever to comprehensiveness. The acupuncture points and symptoms, taken from ancient and modern texts, are primarily selected in accordance with my own personal experience; and I have deliberately exercised self-restraint in order to give priority to clear and speedy location. In considering the few indications I have chosen, may I draw special attention to the above introductory events.

Publication of my work aims to bring this form of therapy closer to those already interested, to encourage beginners to establish this valid and harmless method, and to facilitate progress of their responsible task in this new field of veterinary medicine.

One thing is definite, however, this book cannot be used by anyone as providing a valid excuse for omitting intensive study of the literature on human acupuncture. There he will discover the foundations of ancient thought which will make it possible for him to carry out his work according to the ancient law of harmonizing of all physical processes. From this law it is made clear that the therapeutic influence of acupuncture is principally aimed at changing the functionally disturbed region and less at already degeneratively altered organic states.

I wish all users of this publication good results, together with pleasure in applying acupuncture treatment to horses. I should like to express my thanks to the publishers (B.M.P.) for their praiseworthy co-operation and care in the production of the book.

July 1976   Erwin Westermayer

Acupuncture Method

By the insertion of a needle in a very small clearly delineated skin surface area, acupuncture stimulates a resonance in the body interior. In veterinary medicine, from of old, ways other than needles were known of influencing processes inside the body through stimulation of specific skin areas—I mention here only Moxa, Penetrating or Deep Massage, Friction Massage (for colic), Bathing the limbs, or Blood-letting through incision in the tail.

Since ancient times the Chinese have observed on the skin projection zones of the inner organs and their physiological state, and they have recorded a great number of points and symptoms. Symptoms which are associated with a certain acupuncture point, indicate the choice of site for needling.

The ancient Chinese explained the working of a needle stimulus on a basis which appears quite strange to us, and which I will only briefly indicate here, for a fuller exposition may be studied by a subsequent reading of the widely available literature on human acupuncture. According to this conception the skin points are linked with their related symptoms by a system of vertical pathways, the so-called Meridians. These Meridians or Pathways are named after the organs and systems upon which they mainly work. According to the eastern conception an Energy, in the form of Life-Force, circulates rhythmically in these Meridians. This Life-Force (Ch'i) is bi-polar; yin and yang. These two concepts symbolize positive and negative energy permeating everything living, and whose balance means health and imbalance spells sickness. Needle stimulation at appropriate points can harmonize the circulating Life-Force thereby restoring health.

These ancient ways of thinking will, I admit, not satisfy the western-trained doctor.

Many institutes in both China and the Western World have researched into the working mechanism of acupuncture for many years. As a result, numerous hypotheses and a succession of possible part-explanations have been put forward, the exposition of which would go beyond the limits of this book. I must therefore refer those interested to the literature on the subject. Fundamentally to date we know only that:

a) Veterinary acupuncture has been successfully practised for centuries in China;
b) Veterinary acupuncture can, in many cases, also be of effective assistance to us.

But it has up to now not been possible to demonstrate scientifically how acupuncture works, whether by neural, humoral, or hormonal means.

Acupuncture Points
Characteristics

It is known that an acupuncture point shows itself to be different from its surroundings by differences in sensitivity. It may be more sensitive to pressure and pain, and show a temperature and blood-flow behaviour different from its surroundings. The point re-acting strongly to palpation of the skin and underlying tissue can be assumed to be the Source-position (acupuncture point location).

The horse, through sweat formation on certain parts of the skin, often points out weaknesses of associated organs. Also histologically and chemo-histologically the skin at acupuncture points presents a distinctive picture; electrical skin resistance is lower at these places. On large animals the 'points' are up to the size of a 2p piece. They are frequently found to occur in body surface hollows and depressions, at muscle insertions or above palpable parts of bones or vessels.

Locating Acupuncture Points

Locating acupuncture points on the horse may be done in the following ways:

a) According to topographical-anatomical descriptions;
b) Through palpation and examination of the point for changed sensitivity to pressure and pain, and by the altered state of the Source-point;
c) Through measuring electrical skin-resistance.

There are numerous instruments on the market for the measurement of electrical skin-resistance. Accurate measuring and therewith exact point localisation requires, of course, due consideration of physical facts, such as taking into account the pressure applied to the feeling electrodes, and different skin moisture.

It is self-evident that accurate location of the point is important for therapeutic results.

Types of Needle

Among authors there is no unanimity of needle nomenclature. For example, WEINSTEIN/USA describes the triangular or prism-needle, moxa needle, sharp round needle, the broad-headed needle, etc.

For acupuncture needles, I use canula expendables throughout, as commercially obtainable. Their principal advantage is that they are sterile, cheap and obtainable in various sizes, so that length and strength can be selected according to depth and reaction desired.

Needle Insertion

I favour insertion of the needle with a quick sudden movement and, in the event of the desired depth not being immediately achieved, a slow and sensitive increasing of the depth. Naturally, when needle insertion is being done, due heed must be given to control of the animal, and attention paid to necessary precautions for safeguarding the assistants, the animal, and one's self.

Augmenting Needle Action

Needle action can be augmented by various manipulations of the needle after insertion, these are fully written about in the standard works on human acupuncture. For example, several twirlings of the needle. Needle action augmentation may also be by the so-called 'fire-needle'. This may be used to puncture dense muscle areas, after it has been previously more or less well heated. So too blood-letting at a point is common: in addition to needle action on the point one achieves thereby reticulo-endothelial system stimulation.

Puncture Depth

The depths which I give along with the description of each point can according to my experience only be approximate. The individual build of the animal must always decide the choice of puncture depth.

Horse's Reaction After Needle Insertion

The correct choice and exact location of the point can bring reactions after needle insertion (in Chinese literature these are described as "arrival of the Energy"): for example, drawing in of the flanks, tail erection, muscle relaxation, defacation, and urination. Such reactions are always assessed as favourable signs for a successful outcome. It can be said that, in general, the animal becomes more passive during a needling.

Selection of Points for Treatment

The choice of points to be used can be made following on the examination of the animal, and after the diagnosis finding has been looked up in the symptoms index. However, it is not necessary to needle all the points listed for one symptom, but rather a selection should be made in conformity with the individual data.

I give here as an example "hoof cutis vera inflammation". The Chinese first of all bleed point 77 (this is the place which the veterinary surgeon in this country uses for blood-letting and intravenous injection.) As a distant point the tail-root is needled and likewise bled (143). As regional points, those which lie nearer to the site of the disturbance, one would use, on the forelimbs, points 101, 103, 104, 105, or on the hind limbs, points 137, 139, 140, 141. Some authors also recommend bleeding the lateral and median points 21, 78, 80, 91. In each case the point must be so punctured that blood issues. Then in like manner puncture the points 97, 98, 99, 100, 135, 136, which lie above the lateral and medial digital veins. The more distant points 78 on the vena cephalica humeri and 80 on the vena cephalica accessoria have influence on blood flow through the fore limbs and work on the digestion and metabolism; similarly points 112, 127, 129, 131 on the hind limbs.

Locus–Dolendi Puncture

The so-called 'Locus-dolendi-puncture', puncturing painful points and areas, is the simplest form of acupuncture. This method can be carried out on the horse as the first and simplest measure in all cases of acute swellings resulting from trauma. The swelling is studded with circular or oval rows of needles—I recommend short canula expendables—so that the area looks like a pin cushion. One may expect the swelling to reduce more rapidly than with traditional therapy.

Similar methods may be used in chronic thickening, e.g. carpal tumour. Attention should here be given to the need for repeated needling: two or three times a week to begin with, then once or twice a week until improvement.

It is recommended in the above instances to use in addition the distant points which work on corresponding body areas. Thus one can combine Locus-dolendi-acupuncture and Symptomatic-acupuncture.

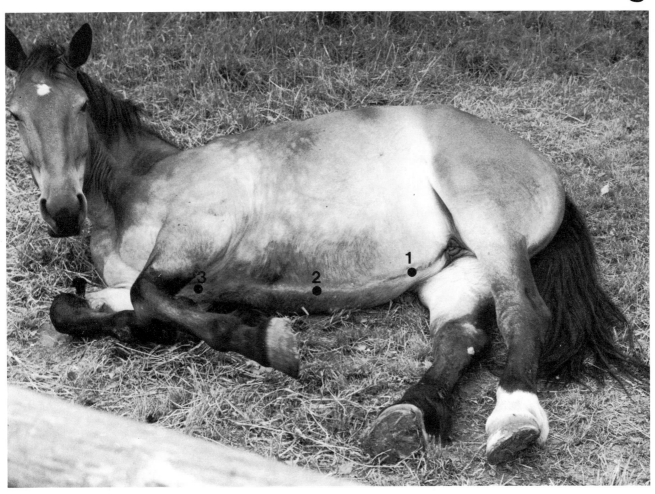

1 Location: Centre of the umbilicus.
   Needle: C. 5—10mm.
   Indications: Facilitation of parturition, sterility.

2 Location: Approximately two handbreadths caudal to the xyphoid process.
   Needle: C. 25—35mm.
   Indications: Stomach disorder, stomach spasm, intestinal colic.

3 Location: Midpoint of the corpus sterni.
   Needle: C. 20—30 mm. Insert needle forwards at an angle.
   Indications: Respiratory tract disorders, emphysema, asthma.

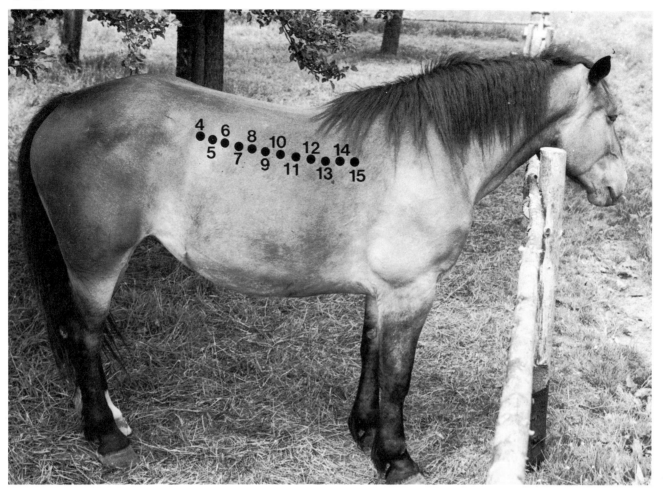

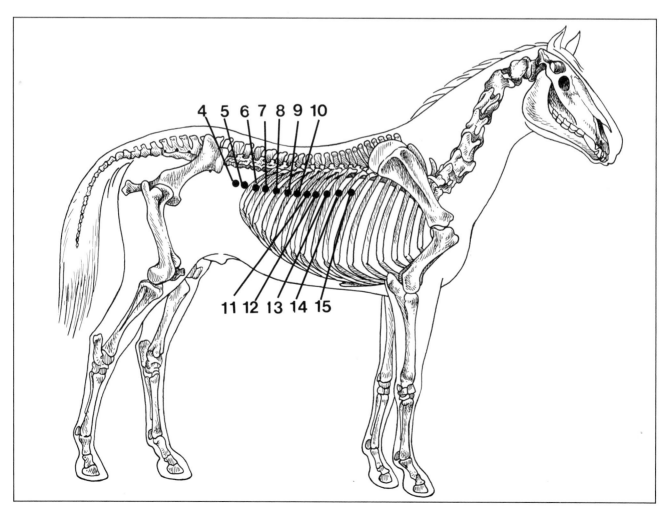

4 Location: Approx. two handbreadths and three fingerwidths below the dorsal ridge, in line with the inter-space between the transverse processes of L.I and L.2, in the iliocostal groove.
  Needle: C. 25—30mm.
  Indications: Intestine inflation, stomach dilatation, constipation, diarrhoea, intestine spasm, pains in the lumbar region, inflammation of the intestines, intestinal rupture.

5 Location: In the body of m. iliocostalis, approximately two handbreadths and three fingerwidths below the dorsal ridge, in line with the interspace between the transverse processes of L.1 and C.18.
  Needle: C. 25—40 mm.
  Indications: Intestine inflation, stomach dilatation, diarrhoea, constipation, intestine spasm, pains in the lumbar region.

6 Location: Approx. two handwidths and three fingerwidths below the dorsal ridge, between C.18 and C.17, in the body of m. iliocostalis.
  Needle: C. 25—30 mm.
  Indications: Indigestion, biliousness, intestine spasm, intestine inflation, enteritis, constipation, gastritis.

7 Location: Approx. two handbreadths and three fingerwidths below the dorsal ridge, between C.17 and C.16, in the body of m. iliocostalis.
  Needle: C. 25—30 mm.
  Indications: Lung dilation, stomach dilatation.

8 Location: Approx. two handbreadths and three fingerwidths below the dorsal ridge, between C.18 and C.17, in the body of m. iliocostalis.
  Needle: C. 25—30 mm.
  Indications: Biliousness, indigestion, intestine spasm, flatulence, stomach dilatation, constipation.

9 Location: Approx. two handbreadths and three fingerwidths below the dorsal ridge, between C.15 and C.14, in the body of m. iliocostalis.
  Needle: C. 25—30 mm.
  Indications: Biliousness, indigestion, intestinal spasm, obstruction (stoppage).

10 Location: Approx. two handbreadths and three fingerwidths below the dorsal ridge, between C.14 and C.13, in the body of the m. iliocostalis.
  Needle: C. 25—30 mm.
  Indications: Indigestion, biliousness, diaphragm disorders, conjunctivitis, keratitis.

11 Location: Approx. two handbreadths and three fingerwidths below the dorsal ridge, between C.13 and C.12, in the body of m. iliocostalis.
  Needle: C. 25—30 mm.
  Indications: Stomach dilation, diaphragm disorders, indigestion, biliousness, flatulence, intestine spasm.

12 Location: Approx. two handbreadths and three fingerwidths below the dorsal ridge, between C.12 and C.11, in the body of m. iliocostalis.
  Needle: C. 25—30 mm.
  Indications: Icterus, constipation, diaphragm disorders, fever, feverish ague, laryngo-pharyngitis, wheezing.

13 Location: Approx. two handbreadths and three fingerwidths below the dorsal ridge, between C.11 and C.10, in the body of m. iliocostalis.
  Needle: C. 25—30 mm.
  Indications: Gastro-enteritis, constipation, lumbago, tracheitis.

14 Location: Approx. two handbreadths and four fingerwidths below the dorsal ridge, between C.10 and C.9, in the body of m. iliocostalis.
  Needle: C. 25—30 mm.
  Indications: Pleuritis, bronchitis, pneumonia, bleeding lungs.

15 Location: Approx. two handbreadths and four fingerwidths below the dorsal ridge, between C.9 and C.8, in the body of m. iliocostalis.
  Needle: C. 25—30 mm.
  Indications: Intestine spasm, overstrain, the staggers, pleuritis, emphysema, generalized spasm.

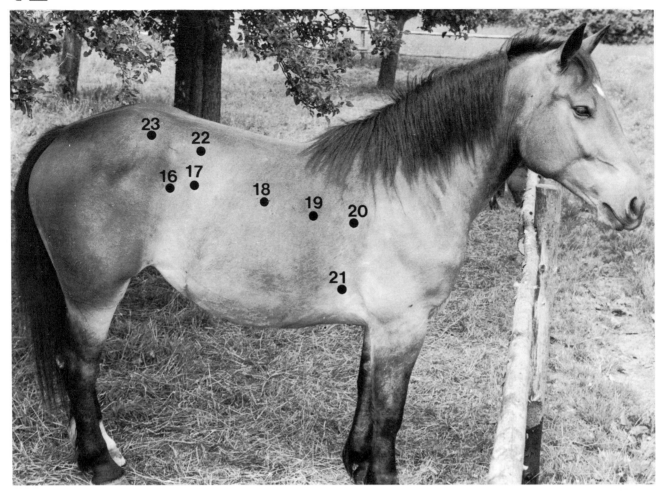

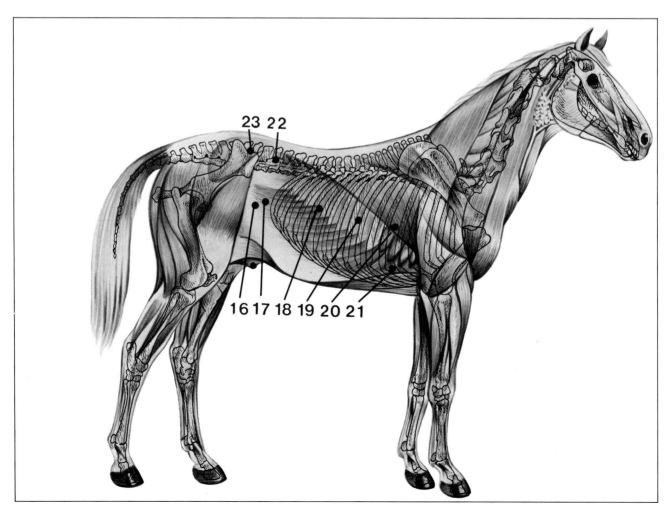

16 Location: Approx. three to four fingerwidths caudal to the costal angle of the last rib.
   Needle: C. 20—25 mm.
   Indications Intestine paralysis, to stimulate peristalsis.

17 Location: Approx. three handbreadths below the dorsal ridge and about a fingerwidth caudal to the last rib.
   NOTE: The point is on the right side only.
   Needle: C. 15—30 mm.
   Indications: Inflammations, colic and inflation of the coecum.

18 Location: Between C.13 and C.14, about three handbreadths and two fingerwidths below the dorsal ridge.
   Needle: C. 15—20 mm.
   Indications: Disturbed functioning of the diaphragm.

19 Location: Between C.9 and C.10, about three handbreadths and two fingerwidths below the dorsal ridge.
   Needle: C. 15—20 mm.
   Indications: Bronchitis, pneumonia, asthma.

20 Location: Between C.6 and C.7. about four handbreadths below the dorsal ridge.
   Needle: C. 15—20 mm.
   Indications: Convulsions, heatstroke, sweating, intestine spasm.

21 Location: Approx. one handbreadth caudal to the point of the elbow, over the vena thoracica interna.
   Needle: C. 6 mm. Bleed.
   Indications: Intestine spasm, heatstroke, fever, stomatitis, inflammation of the hoof and pedal cutis vera, tetanus.

22 Location: At the mid-point of an imaginary vertical line from the caudal edge of the last rib to the dorsal ridge, at the level of the hip protruberance.
   Needle: C. 40—50 mm.
   Indication: Constipation, intestinal colic, flatulence.

23 Location: At the mid-point of an imaginary line from the tuber coxae to the dorsal ridge.
   Needle: C. 40—50 mm.
   Indications: Constipation, intestinal colic, flatulence.

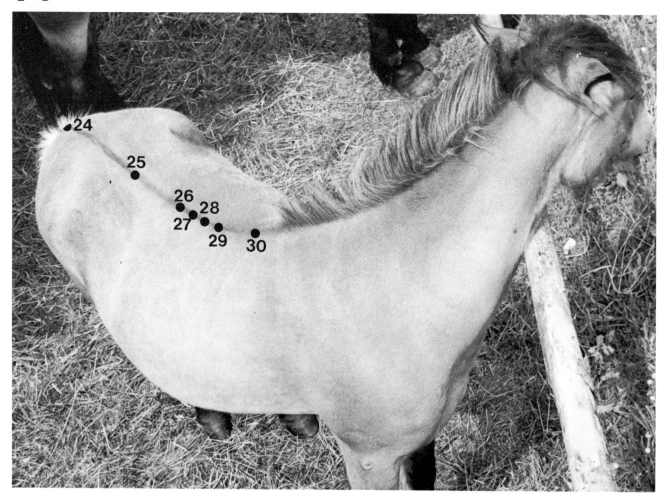

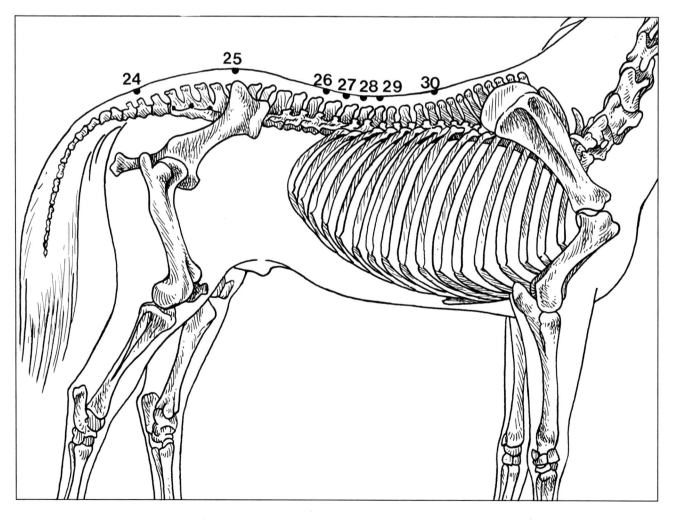

24 Location: On the dorsum of the tail in the depression between the first and second tail vertebrae.
Needle: C. 10 mm.
Indications: Pain in lumbar vertebrae area, hip lameness, lumbago, sterility.

25 Location: In the depression between the spinous processes of L.5 and S.1.
Needle: C. 30—35 mm.
Indications: Hip lameness, pain in lumbar vertebrae area, heatstroke, colic, tetanus, overstrain, feverish shivering.

26 Location: In the depression between the spinous processes of L.1 and L.2.
Needle: C. 10—15 mm.
Indications: Facilitation of parturition, sterility, nephritis.

27 Location: In the depression between the spinous processes of T.18 and L.1.
Needle: C. 10—15 mm.
Indications: Bleeding after castration, epistaxis, haematuria, blood in the stool.

28 Location: In the depression between the spinous processes of T.17 and T.18.
Needle: C. 10—15 mm.
Indications: Bleeding after castration, epistaxis, haematuria, blood in the stool.

29 Location: In the depression between the spinous processes of T.16 and T.17.
Needle: C. 10—15 mm.
Indications: Bleeding after castration, epistaxis, haematuria, blood in the stool.

30 Location: About four fingerwidths behind the withers, between the spinous processes of T.11 and T.12
Needle: C. 10—15 mm.
Indications: Bronchitis, pneumonia, asthma.

N.B. All points on this page are median

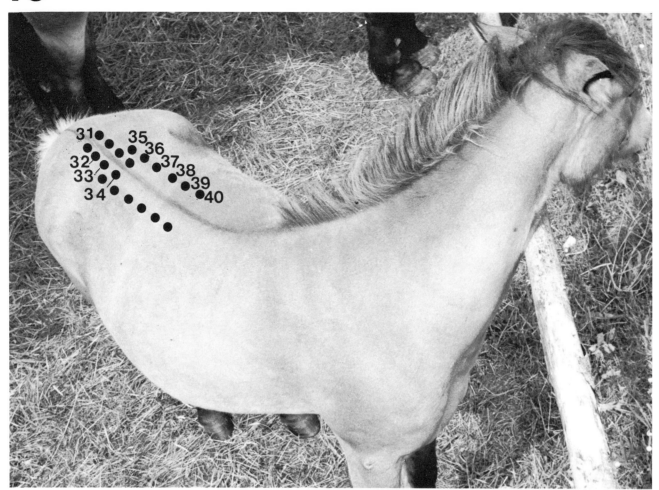

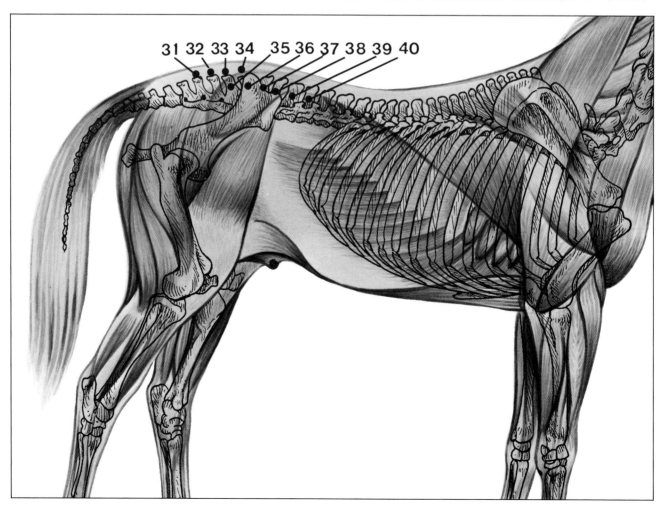

31   Location: Three fingerwidths lateral to the median line, at the level of the interspace between the spinous processes S.4 and S.5, over the sacral foramina.
      Needle: C. 20 mm.
      Indications: To facilitate parturition, hip paralysis, pains and paralysis in lumbar region, pudic nerve paralysis.

32   Location: Three fingerwidths lateral to the median line at the level of the interspace between the spinous processes of S.3 and S.4 over the sacral foramina.
      Needle: C. 20 mm.
      Indications: To facilitate parturition, hip paralysis, pains and paralysis in the lumbar region, pudic nerve paralysis.

33   Location: Three fingerwidths lateral to the median line at the level of the interspace between the spinous processes of S.2 and S.3 over the sacral foramina.
      Needle: C. 20 mm.
      Indications: To facilitate parturition, hip paralysis, pains and paralysis in the lumbar region, pudic nerve paralysis.

34   Location: Three fingerwidths lateral to the median line at the level of the interspace between the spinous processes of S.1 and S.2 over the sacral foramina.
      Needle: C. 20 mm.
      Indications: To facilitate parturition, hip paralysis, pains and paralysis in the lumbar region, pudic nerve paralysis.

35   Location: Approx. one handbreadth lateral to the median line, between the haunch bone and the lateral process of L.6. (Three fingerwidths caudal to Point 36).
      Needle: C. 40–50 mm.
      Indications: Pain and paralysis in lumbar vertebral and sacral region, hip lameness.

36   Location: Approx. one handbreadth lateral to the median line, in the space between L.6 and L.5.
      Needle: C. 30–35 mm.
      Indications: Pain and paralysis in lumbar vertebral and sacral region, hip lameness.

37   Location: Approx. one handbreadth lateral to the median line, in the space between the lateral processes of L.5 and L.4.
      Needle: C. 30 mm.
      Indications: Pains and paralysis in the lumbar vertebral and sacral region, hip lameness.

38   Location: Approx. one handbreadth lateral to the median line, in the space between the lateral processes of L.4 and L.3.
      Needle: C. 35 mm.
      Indications: Pains and paralysis in the lumbar region, lumbago, nephritis, myositis of lumbar musculature.

39   Location: Approx. one handbreadth lateral to the median line, in the space between the lateral processes of L.3 and L.2.
      Needle: C. 35 mm.
      Indications: Pains and paralysis in the lumbar region, lumbago, nepgritis, myositis of lumbar musculature.

40   Location: Approx. one handbreadth lateral to the median line, between the lateral processes of L.2 & L.1
      Needle: C. 35 mm.
      Indications: Pains and paralysis in the lumbar region, lumbago, nephritis, myositis of lumbar musculature.

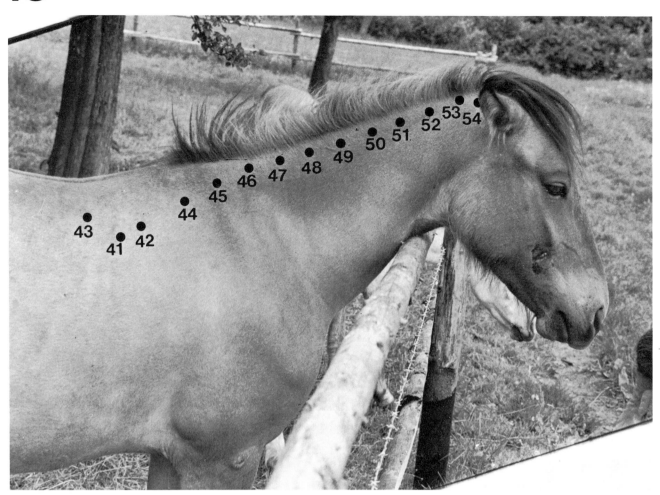

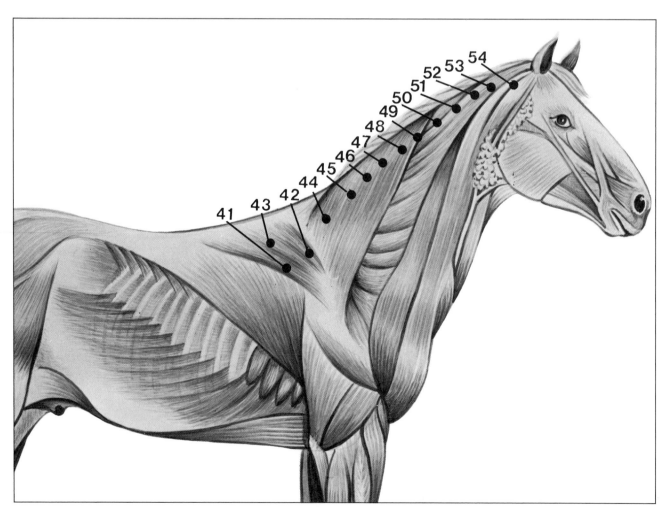

41 Location: Caudal to the scapula, at the junction of the scapula and the scapular cartilage of prolongation.
Needle: Subcutaneous puncture along the posterior border of the scapula, C. 40—60 mm.
Indications: Pain and paresis of n. suprascapularis.

42 Location: Approx. one handbreadth and two fingerwidths below the middle of the superior border of the scapular cartilage of prolongation.
Needle: Puncture subcutaneously at an angle downwards, 80—100 mm.
Indications: Pain and paresis of n. suprascapularis, shoulder joint inflammation, shoulder lameness, shoulder muscle atrophy.

43 Location: About three fingerwidths below the thoracic vertebral spinous processes and two fingerwidths caudal to an imaginary continuation of the line of the scapular spine onto the scapular cartilage of prolongation.
Needle: At an angle downwards caudally, C. 10—15 mm.
Indications: Bronchitis, asthma.

44 Location: Anterior border of the scapula at the junction of the scapula and scapular cartilage of prolongation, in a depression about four fingerwidths below the mane line.
Needle: C. 40—50 mm. along the anterior border of the scapula, slightly downwards.
Indications: Pain and paresis of n.suprascapularis, shoulder lameness, atrophy of shoulder musculature.

45 Location: About two fingerwidths below the mane line and some four fingerwidths anterior to the superior angle of the scapula.
Needle: C. 30—50 mm.
Indications: Tetanus, maladies and pains in the nuchal region, heart weakness, circulation disorders.

46 Location: About two fingerwidths below the mane line at one eighth of the distance along a line joining Point 45 and Point 53.
Needle: C. 30—35 mm.
Indications: Maladies and pains in the nuchal region, tetanus, wheezing.

47 Location: About two fingerwidths below the mane line at two eighths of the distance along a line joining Point 45 and Point 53.
Needle: C. 30—50 mm.
Indications: Maladies and pains in the nuchal region, tetanus.

48 Location: About two fingerwidths below the mane line at three eighths of the distance along a line joining Point 45 and Point 53.
Needle: C. 30—50 mm.
Indications: Maladies and pains in the nuchal region, tetanus.

49 Location: About two fingerwidths below the mane line at four eighths of the distance along a line joining Point 45 and Point 53.
Needle: C. 30—50 mm.
Indications: Maladies and pains in the nuchal region, tetanus.

50 Location: About two fingerwidths below the mane line at five eighths of the distance along a line joining Point 45 and Point 53.
Needle: C. 30—50 mm.
Indications: Maladies and pains in the nuchal region, tetanus.

51 Location: About two fingerwidths below the mane line at six eighths of the distance along a line joining Point 45 and Point 53.
Needle: C. 30—50 mm.
Indications: Maladies and pains in the nuchal region, tetanus, wheezing.

52 Location: About two fingerwidths below the mane line at seven eighths of the distance along a line joining Point 45 and Point 53.
Needle: C. 30—50 mm.
Indications: Maladies and pains in the nuchal region, tetanus, laryngitis, pharyngitis, circulation disorders.

53 Location: About two fingerwidths below the mane line, above the atlas.
Needle: C. 30—50 mm.
Indications: Maladies and pains in the nuchal region, tetanus.

54 Location: Approx. four fingerwidths behind the ear and three fingerwidths lateral to the mane line.
Needle: Puncture at an angle upwards 20—30 mm.
Indications: Tetanus, encephalitis, feverish shivering, pains in the nuchal region.

20

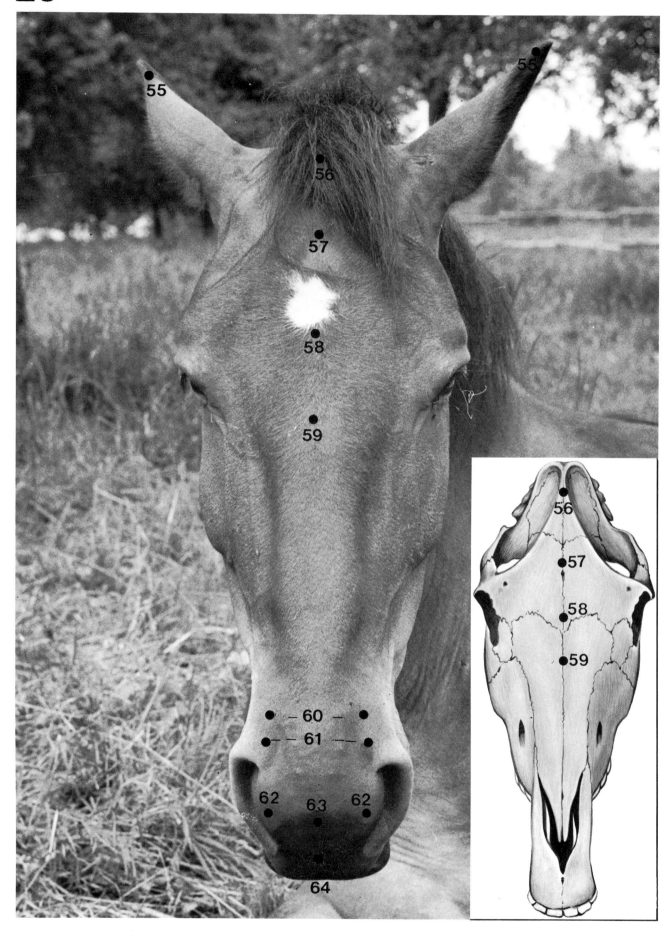

55 Location: Dorsal aspect of the ear at the ear tip on the auricular vein.
Needle: Bleed.
Indications: Abdominal spasm, feverish shivering fever.

56 Location: In the centre of the mane root on the junction line of the left and right external saggital crests of the parietal bone.
Needle: C. 50—60 mm. subcutaneously down towards the nose.
Indications: Tetanus, encephalitis, the staggers, Borna disease.

57 Location: Median line of the head one handbreadth distal to Point 56.
Needle: C. 60—70 mm. subcutaneously down towards the nose.
Indications: Purulent sinusitis, head and lung congestions, tetanus.

58 Location: Where the median line of the head is crossed by the line joining the lateral angles of the eyes.
Needle: Subcutaneously downwards 30 mm. Possibly with heated needles.
Indications: Cerebral haemorrhages, pain in nuchal region.

59 Location: Where the median line of the head is crossed by the line joining the medial angles of the eyes.
Needle: Subcutaneously downwards 50 mm.
Indications: Cerebral haemorrhages, pain in nuchal region.

60 Location: About four fingerwidths above the nostrils, dorsal.
Needle: Subcutaneously sideways towards the septum, bleed.
Indications: Rhinitis, cerebral haemorrhages, lung congestion, overstrain.

61 Location: About two fingerwidths distal to Point 60.
Needle: Subcutaneously sideways towards the septum, bleed.
Indications: Rhinitis, cerebral haemorrhages, lung congestion, overstrain.

62 Location: Upper lip external, on an imaginary line linking the lower part of the nostrils about 5 mm from the nostrils.
Needle: 5 mm.
Indications: Fever, feverish shivering, overstrain.

63 Location: Centre of upper lip at the hair-parting where hair begins.
Needle: C. 10 mm.
Indications: Abdominal spasm, colic.

64 Location: Upper lip external, midway between the borders of the nostrils.
Needle: C. 5 mm.
Indications: Stomatitis, pharyngitis, laryngitis.

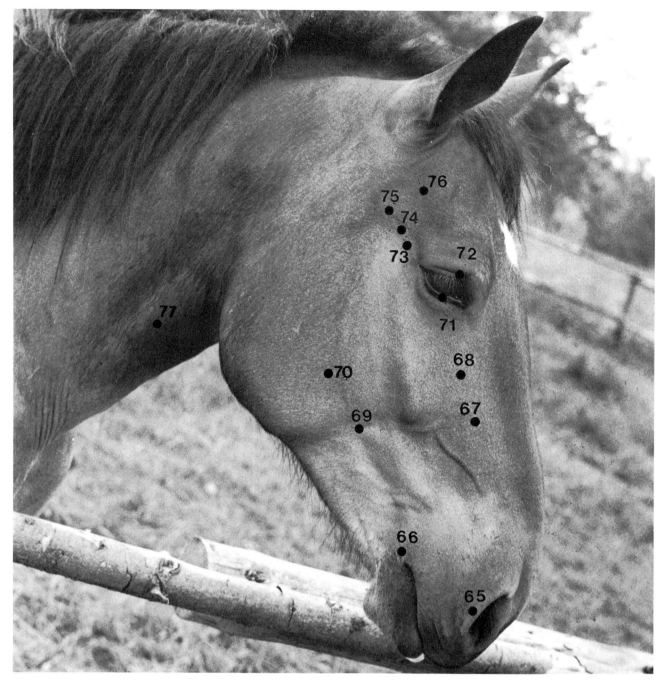

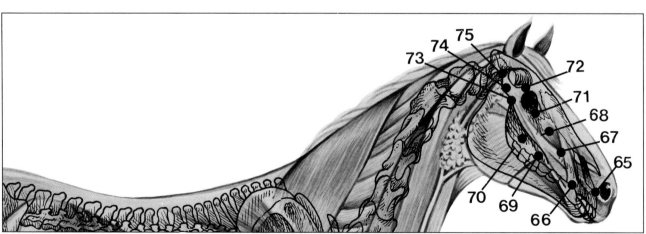

65 Location: At the tip of the nasal alar cartilage.
Needle: C. 5 mm.
Indications: Constipation, abdominal spasm.

66 Location: Outer border of the corner of the mouth, one cm. lateral to the mouth.
Needle: C. 20—30 mm. at an angle inwards.
Indications: Facial nerve paralysis, reduced blood pressure, tetanus.

67 Location: On the vena naso-frontalis some 2 cm below and mouthwards from Point 68.
Needle: C. 5 mm. Bleed.
Indications: Intestinal colic, intestinal inflation, keratitis, constipation, conjunctivitis, recurring eye inflammation.

68 Location: About 25 mm. below the medial angle of the eye, on the vena angularis oculi.
Needle: C. 5—8 mm.
Indications: Intestinal colic, intestinal inflation, constipation, conjunctivitis, keratitis, recurring eye inflammation.

69 Location: Anterior border of the m.masseter, on the extension line from the corner of the mouth to the masseter.
Needle: Subcutaneously C. 60—80 mm. at an angle in the direction of the mouth.
Indications: Tetanus, facial paralysis, affections of the jaw.

70 Location: Approx. four fingerwidths caudal to the anterior border of the masseter, about a handbreadth below the crista facialis, in a depression.
Needle: C. 10 mm. at an angle upwards in the direction of the eye.
Indications: Facial paralysis, masseter spasm, swollen face, bone diseases.

71 Location: On the lower eyelid, at midpoint of the ciliary line.
Needle: Press the eyeball upwards, insert the needle along the upper border of the lacrymal bone, c. 50—60 mm.
Indications: Eye infection, nictitation, lacrimation, recurring eye inflammation.

72 Location: On the upper eyelid, at the midpoint of the ciliary line.
Needle: Press the eyeball downwards, the needle to follow along the border of the zygomatic process about 50 mm.
Indications: Conjunctivitis, keratitis, recurring eye inflammation.

73 Locations: On the vena transversa facii, approx. two fingerwidths behind the lateral angle of the eye.
Needle: C. 30—50 mm. Bleed. Puncture along the vein.
Indications: Conjunctivitis, eye inflammation, facial paresis, heatstroke, fever.

74 Location: On the vena transversa facii, approx. one and a half fingerwidths caudal to Point 73.
Needle: C. 40—60 mm. Bleed.
Indications: Conjunctivitis, eye inflammation, facial paresis, heatstroke, fever.

75 Location: Behind the articulation of the jaw, about three fingerwidths from Point 76 towards the chin.
Needle: C. 40—50 mm, at an angle upwards.
Indications: Tetanus, facial paresis.

76 Location: Above the articulation of the jaw, in the depression under the zygomatic arch.
Needle: C. 10—15 mm, at an angle downwards.
Indications: Tetanus, facial paresis.

77 Location: Between the upper and middle third of the jugular vein. Point for blood-letting.
Needle: As for injection at this place. Bleed.
Indications: Overstrain, heatstroke, brain and lung congestion.

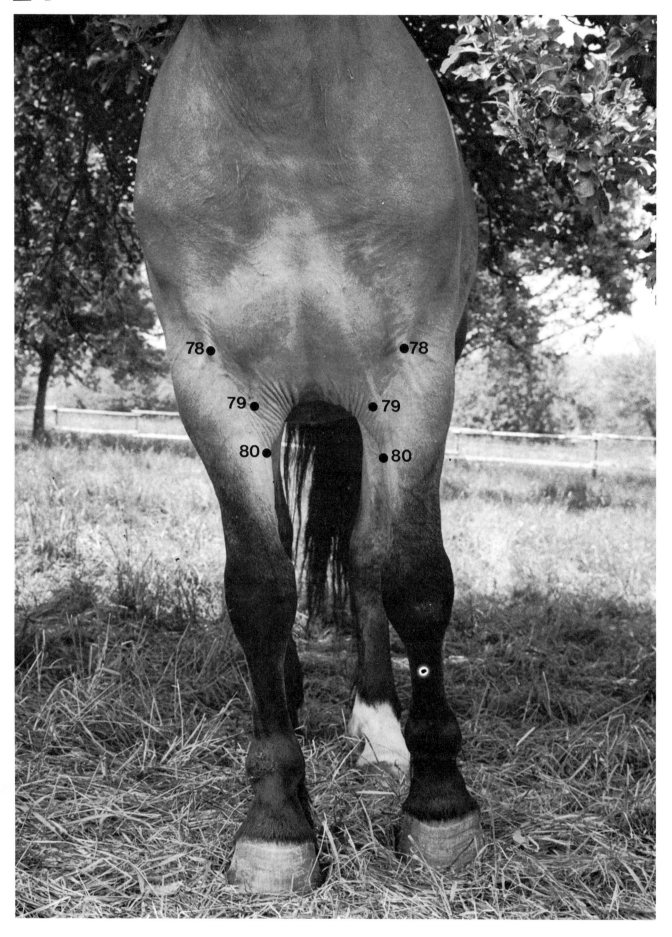

78 Location: At either side of the chest, on the anterior part of the humerus on the vena cephalica humori. The point lies in the lower portion of the lateral furrow between forearm and thorax.
Needle: C. 5 mm. Bleed.
Indications: Shoulder joint and elbow joint inflammation, myositis of chest and humerus musculature, hoof inflammation.

79 Location: In the centre of the muscle groove where the upper part of the forearm and the torso join.
Needle: Sideways in the direction of Point 42, c.140–180 mm (!). Lift the ailing limb, insert needle rapidly. After needle withdrawal shake the leg several times.
Indications: Chronic shoulder lameness, paralysis of n. scapularis.

80 Location: Anterior inner aspect of radius, some 6–8 cm distal to the breastbone, over the vena cephalica accessoria.
Needle: C. 5 mm. Bleed.
Indications: Shoulder and elbow-joint inflammation, myositis of chest and humerus musculature, hoof inflammation, pain in hypogastrium.

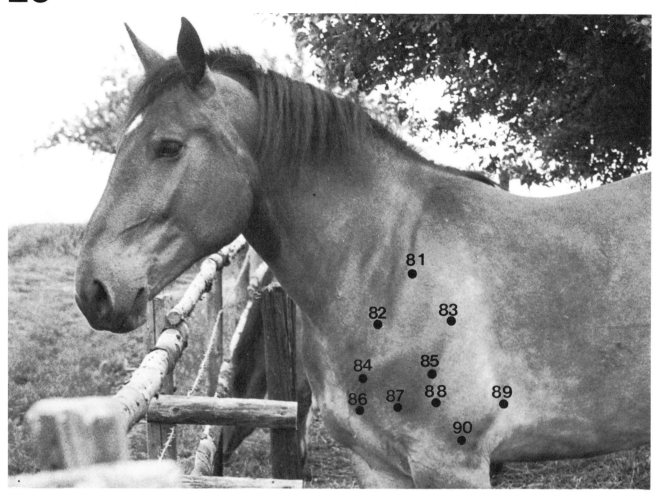

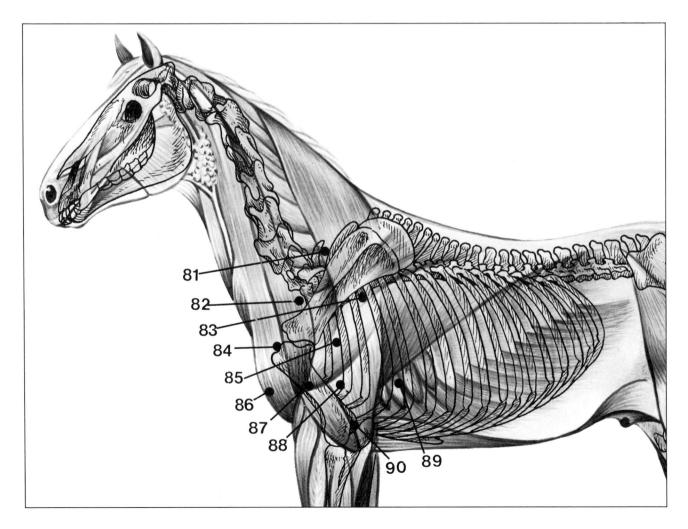

81 Location: Anterior to the scapula in the middle of the nuchal hollow.
Needle: C. 80—100 mm. downwards along the border of the scapula.
Indications: Paralysis of the n. suprascapularis, shoulder lameness, inflammation of the shoulder joint.

82 Location: Anterior border of the scapula, about a handbreadth below Point 81.
Needle: C. 80—100 mm towards the front in the direction of the foot.
Indications: Paralysis of the n. suprascapularis, shoulder lameness, inflammation of shoulder-joint and elbow-joint, myositis of m. sterno-brachio—cephalicus.

83 Location: Posterior border of scapula, about six fingerwidths from the junction of the scapula and the scapular cartilage of prolongation, below Point 41.
Needle: C. 80—100 mm along the caudal edge of scapula in the direction of the shoulder of the same side.
Indications: Shoulder lameness, inflammation of shoulder-joint and elbow-joint, paralysis of n. suprascapularis, myositis of m. sterno-brachiocephalicus.

84 Location: End of the shoulder, at the anterior of the shoulder joint in a depression anterior to the tuberosity of humerus.
Needle: C. 40—50 mm downwards and backwards.
Indications: Shoulder lameness, inflammation of shoulder-joint and elbow-joint, paralysis of n. suprascapularis, myositis of m. sterno-brachiocephalicus.

85 Location: In the muscle groove between m. biceps brachii and m. deltoideus, on the upper border of the m. biceps brachii (caput longum) in a hollow a little above the horizontal level of a line from the throat to the point of the shoulder.
Needle: C. 60—80 mm.
Indications: Myositis of m. sterno-brachiocephalicus, paralysis of n. suprascapularis, shoulder lameness, inflammation of shoulder-joint and elbow-joint.

86 Location: High point of the shoulder in the hollow at the lower border of the tuberosity of humerus.
Needle: C. 20 mm. along the anterior aspect of the humerus inwards and upwards.
Indications: Inflammation of m. sterno-brachiocephalicus, paralysis of n. radialis, shoulder lameness.

87 Location: Posterior aspect of humerus in a depression above the lateral tuberosity of humerus.
Needle: C. 60 mm along the posterior aspect of the humerus, needle at an angle downwards.
Indications: Inflammation of m. sterno-brachiocephalicus, paralysis of n. radialis, shoulder lameness.

88 Location: On the posterior border of the m. deltoideus, in the furrow between the caput longum and caput laterale of m. triceps brachii.
Needle: C. 90—110 mm. Puncture at an angle downwards.
Indications: Inflammation of the joints of the fore limb, paralysis of n. radialis, myositis of chest musculature and of m. brachiocephalicus, heart and circulation disorders, analgesia.

89 Location: In the elbow furrow some two to three fingerwidths above and behind the olecranon process in a depression on the posterior aspect of m. triceps brachii, caput longum, at its lower third.
Needle: C. 10—15 mm.
Indications: Pain and paresis in region of elbow and chest, shoulder and elbow-joint inflammation.

90 Location: Some two fingerwidths below and in front of the point of the elbow, in a depression.
Needle: C. 40—50 mm. perpendicular.
Indications: Paralysis of n. suprascapularis, myositis of chest and throat musculature.

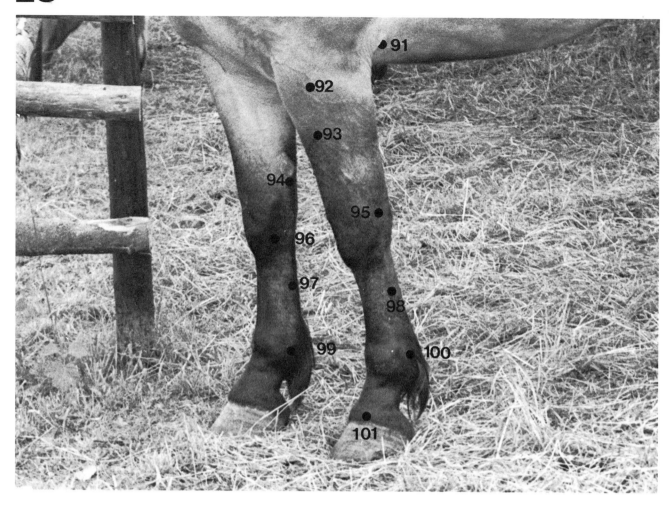

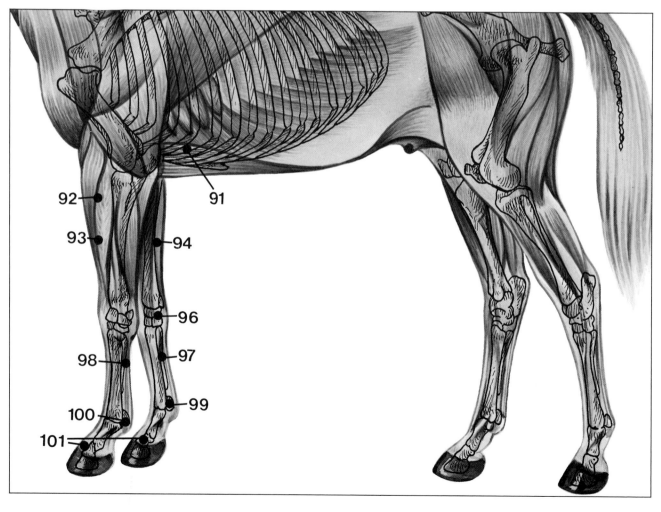

91 Location: In the depression about two fingerwidths below and behind the olecranon process, medially from the elbow to the lower part of the vena thoracica externa.
    Needle: C. 20—25 mm. Puncture from forwards upwards.
    Indications: Pain and paresis in the region of elbow and chest, shoulder- and elbow-joint inflammation.

92 Location: One handbreadth below the elbow-joint in the depression under the lateral tuberosity of the radius, between m. extensor digitorum communis and m. extensor carpi ulnaris.
    Needle: C. 20—30 mm. At an angle forwards.
    Indications: Shoulder lameness, elbow- and carpal-joint inflammation, n. radialis paralysis, myositis of shoulder musculature.

93 Location: About four fingerwidths below Point 92, in a groove between m. extensor carpi radialis and m. extensor digitorum communis.
    Needle: C. 20—30 mm.
    Indications: Tetanus, arthritis of elbow- and carpal-joint, n. radialis paralysis; myositis, tendinitis and tendovaginitis in this area.

94 Location: At junction of middle and distal third of the radius, on the medial aspect of the fore limb, between m. flexor carpi and humeral head of m. flexor carpi ulnaris.
    Needle: C. 10 mm.
    Indications: Heart and circulation deficiency, overstrain, general debility.

95 Location: About two fingerwidths above the lateral aspect of the carpal-joint, in the hollow formed by the posterior border of the radius and the m. flexor digitorum profundus.
    Needle: C. 10 mm. Direction lateral to medial.
    Indications: Carpal-joint inflammation.

96 Location: Medial aspect of the foreleg on the highest part of the carpal-joint, on the vena metacarpi volaris superficialis medialis.
    Needle: C. 3 mm. Bleed.
    Indications: Carpal tumescence (oedema, hygroma, haematoma), infection of carpal-joint, inflammation of the flexor muscles, hoof-joint inflammation.

97 Location: Forefoot medial aspect, between the metacarpus and the medial splint-bone at the proximal quarter of the metacarpus and the proximal third of the splint-bone.
    Needle: C. 5—10 mm.
    Indications: Feverish shivering, fever, recurring eye inflammation, inflammation and swelling in head region, pains in the head and nuchal region, and in the limbs.

98 Location: Forefoot lateral aspect, between the metacarpus and the lateral splint-bone, at about the proximal quarter of the metacarpus and the proximal third of the splint-bone.
    Needle: C. 5—10 mm.
    Indications: Inflammation of the flexor muscles, carpal-joint inflammation, carpal tumescence, hoof-joint inflammation, fetlock-joint inflammation, muscle laceration, atonic constipation.

99 Location: Forefoot medial aspect, on the vena digitalis medialis, at the upper limit of the fetlock-joint.
    Needle: C. 2—3 mm. Bleed.
    Indications: Fetlock-joint contusion, inflammation of fetlock- and carpal-joints, flexor muscle and fetlock-joint inflammation, muscle laceration.

100 Location: Forefoot lateral aspect, on the vena digitalis lateralis, at the upper limit of the fetlock-joint.
    Needle: C. 2—3 mm. Bleed.
    Indications: Fetlock-joint contusion, inflammation of fetlock- and carpal-joints, flexor muscle and fetlock-joint inflammation, muscle laceration.

101 Location: About 1 cm lateral to the midpoint of the anterior coronary band, at the junction of the hairy and hairless integument.
    Needle: C. 7 mm. Bleed.
    Indications: Colic, pedal cutis vera inflammation, hoof- and fetlock-joint inflammation, frog inflammation.

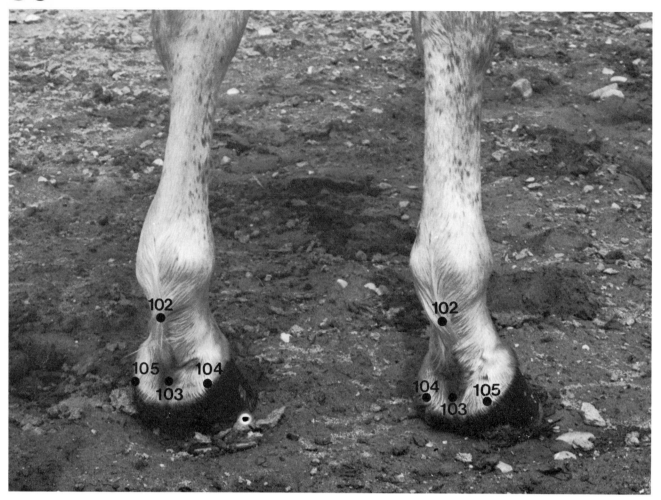

102   Location: In the indentation formed by the sesamoid and the head of the suffraginis on the lower lateral side of the fetlock-joint.

       Needle: C. 5—8 mm.

       Indications: Contusion and inflammation of fetlock-joint, flexor muscle and flexor tendon inflammation, spasm of forefoot musculature.

103   Location: In the centre of the concave surface on the hind part of the hoof, above the frog, at the level of the hoof-joint.

       Needle: With the leg held raised, c. 10—15 mm in the direction of the point of the hoof.

       Indications: Inflammation of the cutis vera, contusion of the coronary articulation, carpal-joint inflammation, muscle laceration, flexor muscle inflammation.

104   Location: In the depression behind the hoof cartilage on the upper border of the frog, medial.

       Needle: C. 7 mm.

       Indications: Cutis vera inflammation, hoof- and fetlock-joint inflammation, frog inflammation.

105   Location: In the depression behind the hoof cartilage on the upper border of the frog, lateral.

       Needle: C. 7 mm.

       Indications: Cutis vera inflammation, frog inflammation, hoof- and fetlock-joint inflammation.

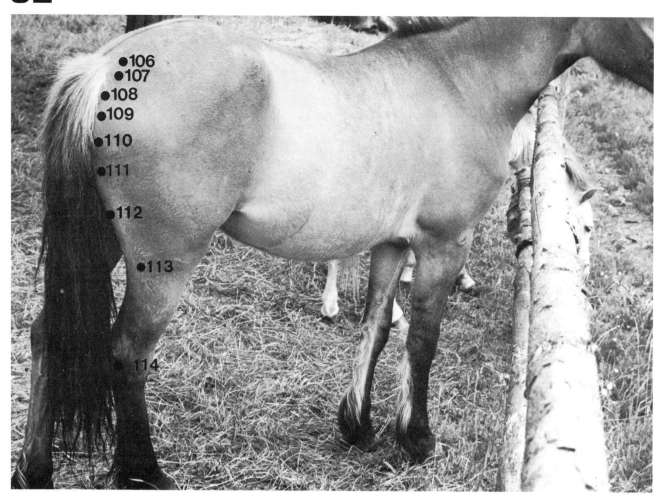

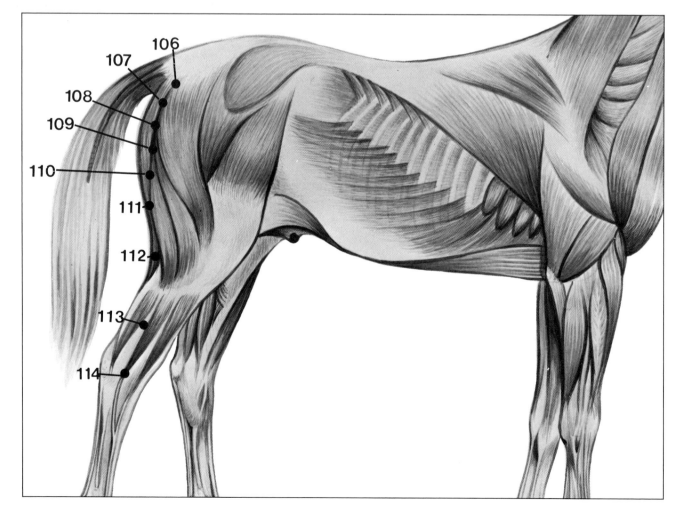

106 Location: Between m. biceps femoris and m. semi-tendinosus at the posterior border of the ischium-bone depression, about four fingerwidths from the dorsal ridge.
Needle: C. 30—40 mm in the direction of the knee of the opposite side.
Indications: Ovary and adnexa malfunction, sterility.

107 Location: Between m. biceps femoris and m. semi-tendinosus caudal border of tuber ischii, about a handbreadth below the dorsal ridge.
Needle: C. 30—40 mm. in the direction of the knee of the opposite side.
Indications: Pudic n. paralysis, anuria, urethraspasm, cystitis, nymphomania, disturbed natural gait rhythm.

108 Location: Lateral to the tail-root, two handbreadths laterally below the dorsal ridge, at the level of the ischium in the muscle groove formed by the m. biceps femoris and the m. semitendinosus.
Needle: C. 50—60 mm.
Indications: Hip-joint inflammation, myositis of mm. biceps femoris, semitendinosus and semimembranosus; paralysis of sacral nerves and femoral nerve.

109 Location: At about a third of the distance along the line joining Point 108 and Point 111.
Needle: C. 50—60 mm.
Indications: Hip-joint inflammation, paralysis of sacral nerves, myositis of mm. biceps femoris, semitendinosus and semimembranosus, paralysis of femoral nerve.

110 Location: Two thirds of the distance along the line joining Point 108 and Point 111.
Needle: C. 50—60 mm.
Indications: Myositis of mm. biceps femoris, semitendinosus, and semimembranosus, hip-joint inflammation, paralysis of sacral nerves and femoral nerve.

111 Location: In the muscle groove between m. biceps femoris and m. semitendinosus, four handbreadths below the dorsal ridge, at the level of the upper limit of the knee-joint.
Needle: C. 50—60 mm.
Indications: Myositis of mm. biceps femoris, semitendinosus and semimembranosus, hip-joint inflammation, paralysis of sacral and femoral nerves.

112 Location: About a handbreadth below Point 111, in the muscle groove between m. semitendinosus and the caudal part of m. biceps femoris, some four fingerwidths above the hollow at the distal end of this muscle, at level of knee-joint.
Needle: C. 40—50 mm.
Indications: Cutis vera inflammation, hip lameness, spasm and paresis of hind limb, skin affections, allergies.

113 Location: Between m. flexor hallucis longus and m. tibialis posticus, about half-way along the tibia, approx. two fingerwidths from the caudal side of the flexor tendon.
Needle: C. 20 mm. at an angle towards the head.
Indications: Stifle-joint inflammation, spasm of lower extremity, bladder spasm, urination disorders, lumbago.

114 Location: At the lower third of a line joining the point of the hock to the external malleolus, and about a fingerwidth below this line.
Needle: C. 30 mm.
Indications: Hock-joint inflammation, cystitis, pains of all kinds. *Caution:* DO NOT puncture in cases of pregnant mares.

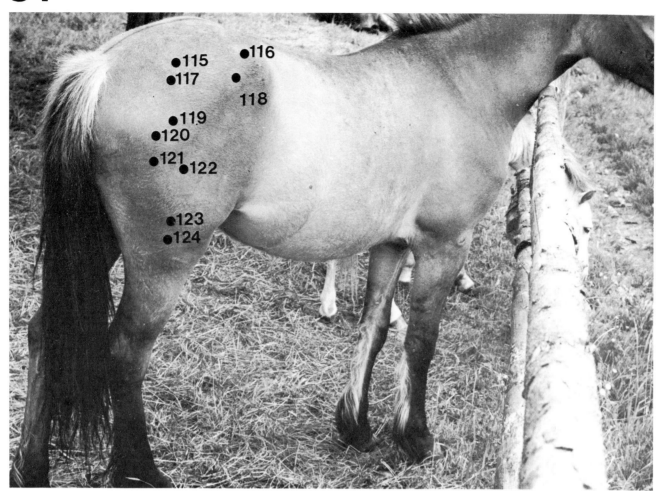

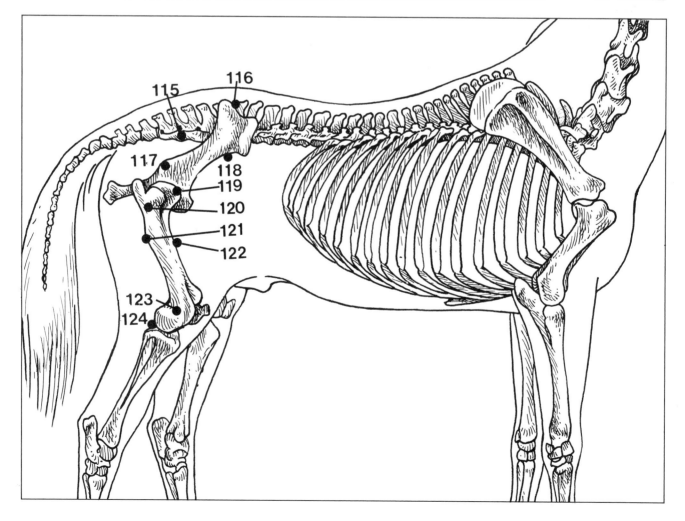

115 Location: In the middle of the line joining the trochanter major pars anterior and Point 25.
Needle: C. 50—60 mm.
Indications: Myositis of hindquarter musculature, especially the biceps femoris; hoof-joint inflammation, paralysis of sacral and femoral nerves.

116 Location: The point lies on an imaginary perpendicular from the tuber coxae to the dorsal ridge, at the junction of the middle and ventral third of this line.
Needle: C. 40—60 mm.
Indications: Myositis of the hip musculature, hip- and knee-joint arthritis; retention, sterility

117 Location: The point lies somewhat above the first third of the line joining Point 25 and the trochanter tertius femoris, or at the mid-point of the line joining Point 118 and the tail-root.
Needle: C. 50—60 mm.
Indications: Liver malfunction, skin affections, hip lameness, inflammation of the sacral nerves, paralysis of n. femoralis.

118 Location: In the depression behind and under the hip protruberance.
Needle: C. 50—70 mm.
Indications: Myositis of hip musculature, hip- and knee-joint arthritis, retention, sterility.

119 Location: In the centre of the depression over the anterior limit of the hip-joint.
Needle: C. 70—80 mm.
Indications: Hip-joint inflammation, pains in hindquarters, paralysis of sacral and femoral nerves, myositis of mm. biceps femoris, semimembranosus, semitendinosus; disturbed gait rhythm.

120 Location: At the centre of the concave area found between the trochanter major and trochanter tertius femoris, anterior to the edge of the bone.
Needle: C. 30 mm.
Indications: Hip-joint inflammation, pains in hindquarters, paralysis of nn. femoralis, tibialis, and fibularis.

121 Location: In the depression behind and below the trochanter tertius femoris.
Needle: C. 50—60 mm.
Indications: Pains in the hindquarters, Myositis of m. biceps femoris, paralysis of nn. femoralis, tibialis, fibularis; nephritis, lumbago, anuria, urination disorders.

122 Location: At midpoint of a line joining the anterior border of the great trochanter and the patella.
Needle: C. 30—40 mm.
Indications: Myositis of hip and upper thigh musculature, hindquarter pains, hip- and knee-joint inflammation.

123 Location: Behind the knee-joint in a depression at the upper border of the lateral epicondyle.
Needle: C. 50—60 mm.
Indications: Arthritis of knee-joint; constipation, gastroenteritis, hindquarter pains.

124 Location: Behind the knee-joint, in a depression at the posterior distal extremity of the lateral tibial condyle.
Needle: C. 50—60 mm.
Indications: Hock-joint inflammation; paralysis of n. tibialis and n. fibularis; hindquarter pains.

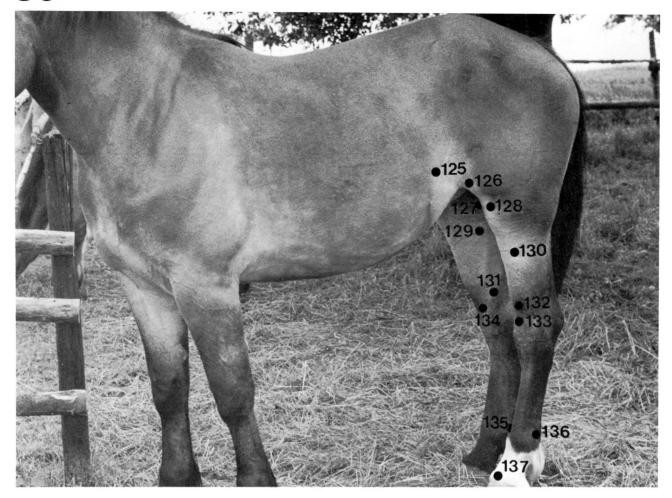

●125
●126
127 ●128
129●
●130
131 ●
●132
134 ● ●133
135 ●136
137●

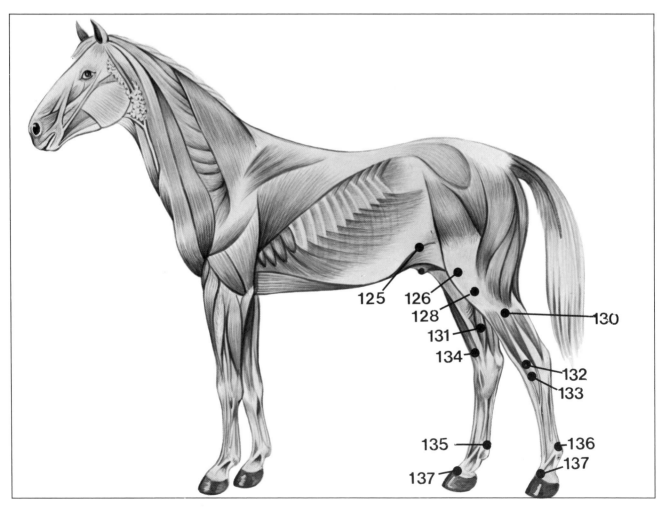

125
126
128
130
131
134
132
133
135 136
137 137

125 Location: About a handbreadth above the knee-fold and four fingerwidths cranially from the edge of the m. tensor fasciae latae.
Needle: C. 10–20 mm.
Indications: Bladder spasm, urethra spasm, anuria, urination disorders, lumbago.

126 Location: In the depression above the patella.
Needle: C 10–20 mm.
Indications: Knee-joint inflammation, pains in hind limb.

127 Location: Inner aspect of the thigh, on the vena saphena, some five fingerwidths below the midpoint where thigh and torso join.
Needle: C. 5 mm. DO NOT PUNCTURE THE VEIN.
Indications: Inflammation of hip- and knee-joints, myositis of mm. semitendinosus and biceps femoris, cutis vera inflammation; orchitis, oedema of scrotum and lower extremity after castration.

128 Location: Lower border of patella, between the lateral and medial ligaments.
Needle: C. 10–20 mm.
Indications: Knee-joint inflammation, pain in hind limb, tendovaginitis, paralysis of n. femoralis, n. tibialis and n. fibularis.

129 Location: About four fingerwidths below Point 127.
Needle: C. 5 mm.
Indications: Inflammation of hip- and knee-joints, myositis of mm. semitendinosus, semimembranosus and biceps femoris; cutis vera inflammation, orchitis, oedema of scrotum and lower extremity after castration.

130 Location: In the muscle triangle formed between m. extensor digitalis longus and m. extensor pedis lateralis on the lateral ligament. The Point lies in a depression below the head of the fibula.
Needle: C. 20 mm.
Indications: Arthritis of knee- and hock-joint, paralysis of n. tibialis and n. fibularis; disorders consequent on stomach functioning deficiency; general toning point, gastroenteritis, colic.

131 Location: Medial lower segment of the leg, between m. flexor digitalis longus and m. tibialis posticus where they become sinewy, on the subjacent portion of the m. flexor hallucis longus, about three fingerwidths from the caudal border of the flexor tendon.
Needle: C. 10–20 mm. Puncture latero-ventrally.
Indications: Sterility, facilitation of parturition, cutis vera inflammation, haemorrhagic disorders of hind limb, allergy, liver deficiency, nymphomania, constipation.

132 Location: Two fingerwidths above Point 133 in a depression formed by the lower border of the external malleolus.
Needle: C. 3 mm.
Indications: Metatarsal-joint inflammation, flexor tendon inflammation, paralysis of n. fibularis and n. tibialis.

133 Location: On the concave surface over the vena saphena superficialis ramus cranialis, at the level of the metatarsal-joint.
Needle: C. 3 mm. Bleed.
Indications: Hock-joint inflammation, flexor tendon inflammation.

134 Location: Anterior inferior aspect of tibia, between the medial and lateral malleoli, approx. one fingerwidth medial to the mid-line.
Needle: C. 5 mm.
Indications: Metatarsal-joint inflammation, paralysis of n. fibularis and n. tibialis.

135 Location: On the vena digitalis medialis, at the upper border of the fetlock-joint.
Needle: C. 3 mm. Bleed congested vein.
Indications: Contusion of fetlock- and hock-joints, tendon and tendon sheath inflammation.

136 Location: On the vena digitalis lateralis, at the upper border of the fetlock-joint.
Needle: C. 3 mm Bleed congested vein.
Indications: Contusion of fetlock- and hock-joints, tendon and tendon sheath inflammation.

137 Location: Anterior centre of coronary band (hind hoof) at the junction of hairy and hairless integument.
Needle: C. 3–5 mm. Bleed.
Indications: Cutis vera inflammation, inflammation of frog and sole of foot, os coronae articulation inflammation, colic, constipation.

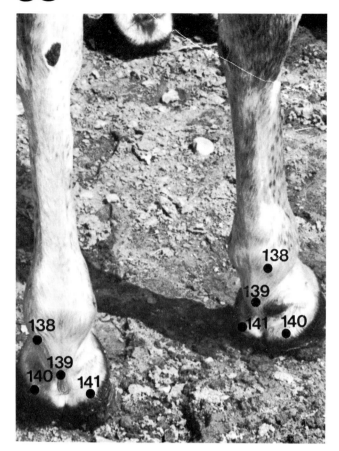

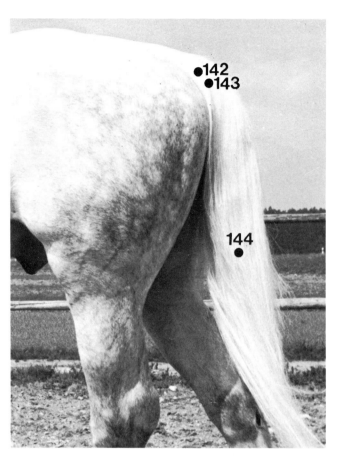

138 Location: In the indentation below the sesamoid bone, on the lateral part of the fetlock-joint.
    Needle: C. 5—8 mm.
    Indications: Contusion and inflammation of fetlock-joint, flexor muscle and flexor tendon inflammation, spasm of hind-foot musculature.

139 Location: In the midpoint of the concavity at the posterior of the hoof, above the frog, at the level of the pedal-joint.
    Needle: C. 10—15 mm. With the leg raised, puncture in the direction of the point of the hoof.
    Indications: Cutis vera inflammation, contusion of os coronae articulation, hock-joint inflammation, muscle laceration, flexor muscle inflammation.

140 Location: In the depression behind the hoof cartilage, at the upper border of the frog, lateral.
    Needle: C. 7 mm.
    Indications: Hoof-joint and fetlock-joint inflammation, cutis vera inflammation, frog inflammation.

141 Location: In the depression behind the foot cartilage at the upper border of the frog, medial.
    Needle: C. 7 mm.
    Indications: Hoof-joint and fetlock-joint inflammation, cutis vera inflammation, frog inflammation.

142 Location: In the hollow between anus and tail vertebrae.
    Needle: C. 80 mm. Tail held up, puncture parallel to the tail root.
    Indications: Facilitation of parturition, colic, diarrhoea, constipation, rectal paralysis, anal fissure, pruritis ani, vaginitis.

143 Location: With the tail pressed up high, about four fingerwidths from the tail root towards the tail, on the underside of the tail.
    Needle: C. 5 mm. Bleed.
    Indications: Constipation, pains in lumbar and sacral region.

144 Location: At the tip of the tail, at the last vertebra.
    Needle: C. 7—10 mm.
    Indications: Overstrain, heatstroke, feverish shivering, fever, cerebral hyperaemia, cerebral anaemia, poisoning, allergy.

Indications and Symptoms Index